This food diary belongs to:

Name   :_______________

Address   :_______________

____

____

Phone #   :_______________________________

Email add   :_______________________________

In case of emergency,
pls. call any of the following:

Contact 1
Name   :_______________________________
Phone #   :_______________________________

Contact 2
Name   :_______________________________
Phone#   :_______________________________

Contact 3
Name   :_______________________________
Phone #   :_______________________________

How to use this food diary:

1. Record date, time, and amount of food, beverage, medicine, and supplement intake on the space provided.

2. If a symptom or unusual reaction to the intake occurs, record time of occurrence, symptom or a detailed observation, and level of symptom.

   i)   Symptoms may include:
   -rash;
   -itching of eyes and face;
   -congestion or difficulty of breathing;
   -hives;
   -abdominal cramps;
   -vomiting; and
   -dizziness;

   ii)   Level of symptom may be classified into:
   -Mild (ex: localized itching)
   -Moderate (ex: itching that occurs in more than 1 part of the body)
   -Severe (swelling and difficulty in breathing)

3. If possible, avoid consuming, in a day, more than 1 type food, beverage, medicine, or supplement that you think you are possibly allergic to. This is

in order to avoid confusing results on which intake caused a symptom.

4. DISCLAIMER. This food diary is not intended for self-diagnosis but to assist you on your doctor's visit to discuss a medical condition which may or may not be related to food, beverage, and medicine or supplement allergy.

This is helpful for breastfeeding moms, and those who are suffering from eczema, allergic asthma, recurring rash or hives, and other allergy related illnesses.

DATE	TIME	FOOD, BEVERAGE, MEDICINE, AND SUPPLEMENT	AMT

TIME	SYMPTOM / OBSERVATION	LEVEL

DATE	TIME	FOOD, BEVERAGE, MEDICINE, AND SUPPLEMENT	AMT

TIME	SYMPTOM / OBSERVATION	LEVEL

DATE	TIME	FOOD, BEVERAGE, MEDICINE, AND SUPPLEMENT	AMT

TIME	SYMPTOM / OBSERVATION	LEVEL

DATE	TIME	FOOD, BEVERAGE, MEDICINE, AND SUPPLEMENT	AMT

TIME	SYMPTOM / OBSERVATION	LEVEL

DATE	TIME	FOOD, BEVERAGE, MEDICINE, AND SUPPLEMENT	AMT

TIME	SYMPTOM / OBSERVATION	LEVEL

DATE	TIME	FOOD, BEVERAGE, MEDICINE, AND SUPPLEMENT	AMT

TIME	SYMPTOM / OBSERVATION	LEVEL

DATE	TIME	FOOD, BEVERAGE, MEDICINE, AND SUPPLEMENT	AMT

TIME	SYMPTOM / OBSERVATION	LEVEL

DATE	TIME	FOOD, BEVERAGE, MEDICINE, AND SUPPLEMENT	AMT

TIME	SYMPTOM / OBSERVATION	LEVEL

DATE	TIME	FOOD, BEVERAGE, MEDICINE, AND SUPPLEMENT	AMT

TIME	SYMPTOM / OBSERVATION	LEVEL

DATE	TIME	FOOD, BEVERAGE, MEDICINE, AND SUPPLEMENT	AMT

TIME	SYMPTOM / OBSERVATION	LEVEL

DATE	TIME	FOOD, BEVERAGE, MEDICINE, AND SUPPLEMENT	AMT

TIME	SYMPTOM / OBSERVATION	LEVEL

DATE	TIME	FOOD, BEVERAGE, MEDICINE, AND SUPPLEMENT	AMT

TIME	SYMPTOM / OBSERVATION	LEVEL

DATE	TIME	FOOD, BEVERAGE, MEDICINE, AND SUPPLEMENT	AMT

TIME	SYMPTOM / OBSERVATION	LEVEL

DATE	TIME	FOOD, BEVERAGE, MEDICINE, AND SUPPLEMENT	AMT

TIME	SYMPTOM / OBSERVATION	LEVEL

DATE	TIME	FOOD, BEVERAGE, MEDICINE, AND SUPPLEMENT	AMT

TIME	SYMPTOM / OBSERVATION	LEVEL

DATE	TIME	FOOD, BEVERAGE, MEDICINE, AND SUPPLEMENT	AMT

TIME	SYMPTOM / OBSERVATION	LEVEL

DATE	TIME	FOOD, BEVERAGE, MEDICINE, AND SUPPLEMENT	AMT

TIME	SYMPTOM / OBSERVATION	LEVEL

DATE	TIME	FOOD, BEVERAGE, MEDICINE, AND SUPPLEMENT	AMT

TIME	SYMPTOM / OBSERVATION	LEVEL

DATE	TIME	FOOD, BEVERAGE, MEDICINE, AND SUPPLEMENT	AMT

TIME	SYMPTOM / OBSERVATION	LEVEL

DATE	TIME	FOOD, BEVERAGE, MEDICINE, AND SUPPLEMENT	AMT

TIME	SYMPTOM / OBSERVATION	LEVEL

DATE	TIME	FOOD, BEVERAGE, MEDICINE, AND SUPPLEMENT	AMT

TIME	SYMPTOM / OBSERVATION	LEVEL

DATE	TIME	FOOD, BEVERAGE, MEDICINE, AND SUPPLEMENT	AMT

TIME	SYMPTOM / OBSERVATION	LEVEL

DATE	TIME	FOOD, BEVERAGE, MEDICINE, AND SUPPLEMENT	AMT

TIME	SYMPTOM / OBSERVATION	LEVEL

DATE	TIME	FOOD, BEVERAGE, MEDICINE, AND SUPPLEMENT	AMT

TIME	SYMPTOM / OBSERVATION	LEVEL

DATE	TIME	FOOD, BEVERAGE, MEDICINE, AND SUPPLEMENT	AMT

TIME	SYMPTOM / OBSERVATION	LEVEL

DATE	TIME	FOOD, BEVERAGE, MEDICINE, AND SUPPLEMENT	AMT

TIME	SYMPTOM / OBSERVATION	LEVEL

DATE	TIME	FOOD, BEVERAGE, MEDICINE, AND SUPPLEMENT	AMT

TIME	SYMPTOM / OBSERVATION	LEVEL

DATE	TIME	FOOD, BEVERAGE, MEDICINE, AND SUPPLEMENT	AMT

TIME	SYMPTOM / OBSERVATION	LEVEL

DATE	TIME	FOOD, BEVERAGE, MEDICINE, AND SUPPLEMENT	AMT

TIME	SYMPTOM / OBSERVATION	LEVEL

DATE	TIME	FOOD, BEVERAGE, MEDICINE, AND SUPPLEMENT	AMT

TIME	SYMPTOM / OBSERVATION	LEVEL

DATE	TIME	FOOD, BEVERAGE, MEDICINE, AND SUPPLEMENT	AMT

TIME	SYMPTOM / OBSERVATION	LEVEL

DATE	TIME	FOOD, BEVERAGE, MEDICINE, AND SUPPLEMENT	AMT

TIME	SYMPTOM / OBSERVATION	LEVEL

DATE	TIME	FOOD, BEVERAGE, MEDICINE, AND SUPPLEMENT	AMT

TIME	SYMPTOM / OBSERVATION	LEVEL

DATE	TIME	FOOD, BEVERAGE, MEDICINE, AND SUPPLEMENT	AMT

TIME	SYMPTOM / OBSERVATION	LEVEL

DATE	TIME	FOOD, BEVERAGE, MEDICINE, AND SUPPLEMENT	AMT

TIME	SYMPTOM / OBSERVATION	LEVEL

DATE	TIME	FOOD, BEVERAGE, MEDICINE, AND SUPPLEMENT	AMT

TIME	SYMPTOM / OBSERVATION	LEVEL

DATE	TIME	FOOD, BEVERAGE, MEDICINE, AND SUPPLEMENT	AMT

TIME	SYMPTOM / OBSERVATION	LEVEL

DATE	TIME	FOOD, BEVERAGE, MEDICINE, AND SUPPLEMENT	AMT

TIME	SYMPTOM / OBSERVATION	LEVEL

DATE	TIME	FOOD, BEVERAGE, MEDICINE, AND SUPPLEMENT	AMT

TIME	SYMPTOM / OBSERVATION	LEVEL

DATE	TIME	FOOD, BEVERAGE, MEDICINE, AND SUPPLEMENT	AMT

TIME	SYMPTOM / OBSERVATION	LEVEL

DATE	TIME	FOOD, BEVERAGE, MEDICINE, AND SUPPLEMENT	AMT

TIME	SYMPTOM / OBSERVATION	LEVEL

DATE	TIME	FOOD, BEVERAGE, MEDICINE, AND SUPPLEMENT	AMT

TIME	SYMPTOM / OBSERVATION	LEVEL

DATE	TIME	FOOD, BEVERAGE, MEDICINE, AND SUPPLEMENT	AMT

TIME	SYMPTOM / OBSERVATION	LEVEL

DATE	TIME	FOOD, BEVERAGE, MEDICINE, AND SUPPLEMENT	AMT

TIME	SYMPTOM / OBSERVATION	LEVEL

DATE	TIME	FOOD, BEVERAGE, MEDICINE, AND SUPPLEMENT	AMT

TIME	SYMPTOM / OBSERVATION	LEVEL

DATE	TIME	FOOD, BEVERAGE, MEDICINE, AND SUPPLEMENT	AMT

TIME	SYMPTOM / OBSERVATION	LEVEL

DATE	TIME	FOOD, BEVERAGE, MEDICINE, AND SUPPLEMENT	AMT

TIME	SYMPTOM / OBSERVATION	LEVEL

DATE	TIME	FOOD, BEVERAGE, MEDICINE, AND SUPPLEMENT	AMT

TIME	SYMPTOM / OBSERVATION	LEVEL

DATE	TIME	FOOD, BEVERAGE, MEDICINE, AND SUPPLEMENT	AMT

TIME	SYMPTOM / OBSERVATION	LEVEL

DATE	TIME	FOOD, BEVERAGE, MEDICINE, AND SUPPLEMENT	AMT

TIME	SYMPTOM / OBSERVATION	LEVEL

REMINDERS